How to Prevent Stretch Marks During Maternity and Bring Sexy Back After Pregnancy

The Best Way to Remove Stretch Mark and Be Pregnancy Safe for the Baby

Lili Bloggs

Table of Contents

Chapter 1:
Introduction

My name is Lora; I am a junior executive in a traveling agency. I am an only child.

I grew up feeling all the love from my parents. My parents passed away in a car accident recently. My father is

I am at the peak of my career, and I am an excellent and responsible woman. I just had my birthday, and I turned 28.

I got pregnant a year ago, and it is a blessing because my boyfriend and I got married a year before that. It feels like we have been waiting for it for a long time.

I had the most beautiful wedding, with family and close friends. It was a dream wedding, with the most beautiful gown and a lovely prince—the honeymoon trip in the Bahamas, the most luxurious of all.

I usually travel, and to my delight, I always wear what I like. Two of my best assets are my legs and my flawless skin. Working in a traveling agency, I must look good wearing corporate mini dresses.

I am exposed to different types of people, dealing with customers and big bosses of big companies. I love my job, and it has an excellent opportunity to meet different kinds of people.

That's how I met my man. He is handsome and a successful Veterinarian.

I had many suitors during my single years, but gladly I picked the best man of them all. His name is Richard, a half-American/ Irish man whom I adore dearly. A good cook and a very sensible man who loves me.

He has a big family and the most wonderful mother of all. Always has an answer to everything. I still remember when I was six months pregnant; she talked about stretch marks and kept telling me to be careful, but during that time, I was in a bubble where I thought I was the most beautiful woman in the world.

My husband always kept telling me that until I woke up to the reality that I had stretch marks all over my belly and legs.

Having twins in my belly is very overwhelming. I never give any attention until it grows bigger and bigger. Although I already noticed how my belly is too big and the skin is super stretchy, I didn't mind at all.

I feel bad not listening to my mother-in-law and taking her advice about it. My doctor even gave me the idea about it, but it didn't bother me until that day came when I saw how bad it looked.

It is like something hard hit me and made me realize that it's all my fault and too late.

Don't lose hope to all the women out there who suffer from stretch marks, are newly mothers, and got pregnant with more than one. You can still get rid of the nasty stretch marks in your body.

Even though these are most common to mothers, some teenagers also suffer from this kind of problem. It is also common for young girls and boys to lose and to gain weight can also be one of the reasons for having stretch marks.

Chapter 2:
How I Got My First Stretch Marks

I remember the first time I got pregnant and how happy it made me. My dream had finally come true after years of wanting one so bad. But now that my body changes in ways you can't see or feel, it doesn't quite match up anymore for some reason?

The joys of being a mother are overwhelming, but some worries come in between the happy moments. You only want what's suitable for your kids, and sometimes you forget about yourself and then realize that later on, and for me, I thought it was too late.

My husband still comes home from work every day, telling me he loves sexy womanhood as always. Still, there's just something different when all this new skin starts showing up on his side of things while mine remains cocooned throughout six months with nothing else changing except weight gain/loss (which isn't always indicative).

I tried to cover up the first stretch marks on my inner thighs, but it just wasn't enough. It happened after long hours at work one day, and there was nothing I could do about them then either because you have time before pregnancy when things are happening slower than during pregnancy where every second counts!

My husband encouraged me and told me that it was no big deal; he loves my body. He keeps on telling me that I even look good now and glowing in so many ways. It somehow makes me uncomfortable.

No matter what he says, the fact is that I can see them, and the reality is; I couldn't stop them- the stretch marks on my inner thighs became redder with each day until they were pink with some blue dots here and there.

However, it is not surprising that a lot of pregnant women worry about their stretch marks. The idea is too much for them, too many worries, too much responsibility, and it can be pretty challenging to find clothes that will not show them off.

This problem is common to working mothers like me. We share the same worries that someone might notice or our husband might find it unappealing. Yes, it may not be a big deal to some, but I took it very seriously. I want my husband to still look at me the same way when we got married. I want to look good for him and for myself too.

Having flawless skin is very appealing for me, and before I got pregnant, I always had the need to take care of my skin and my body. It is one of my best assets, you know; my young, flawless skin and my body go with it too.

Most of us are not well informed about the effects of pregnancy. So, I think you have to take these topics seriously and not the other way around. Pregnancy and health must be protected against potential complications wherein both mother and child undergo modifications to minimize risk factors such as smoking or excessive exercise during pregnancy.

During pregnancy with my twins, I got stretch marks on my legs, and they looked like silver lines when the sun hit them just right. After incubation, it took me a long time to prevent my stretch marks from becoming shiny. Yes, we can find ways to hide these marks, but some are peaking through our clothes and can be very noticeable. I'm not too fond of the way it looks; it looks horrible.

I took the liberty of exercising after pregnancy, such as walking, prenatal yoga, Pilates, weights, jogging, and swimming. I want to get back to my feet and look precisely the same way I was. I also eat healthy foods and take time to pamper myself once in a while. I told myself, I have to take care of myself, my husband, and my family.

I am a young wife and new mom. My two daughters were born just five months ago, but people are already telling me to prevent getting stretch marks again! Many of them even told me not to do this time around for my skin's health- which is frustrating because I'm struggling with guilt from the last ones that stretch marks didn't stop before they happened all over again. It became a pressure for me that all I did was worry about it.

Before giving birth, my husband and I used to go out and have a fancy dinner, I used to wear sexy mini dresses, and I always captivated His attention. They were there before, but at least I had time to get used to them. Now it seems like I have many concerns about it. I am struggling to find ways to deal with it.

Getting stretch marks is not a nice thing to see. I sometimes can't wear the old outfits that I used to love. I used to have flawless skin, especially in my legs, and I know He loves how it looks. I love the way I look, but now it seems that it gives me too much stress not to wear my old outfits.

Last night, my husband took me out to dinner. I was so glad to find a sitter at the last moment, and I was so excited because we finally had to go out and enjoy ourselves. I was so happy to find the best outfit because it had been a long time. I want to look good for my husband, and I want to look good for myself.

Finally, I found the best red dress that looked like a knockout. I am getting ready, and because I felt happy, I almost forgot about the stretch marks on my lower leg.

I hurriedly took a shower and put on the lovely dress; as I gazed at myself in the mirror as I was putting some makeup on, there it was peeking at me. I felt so frustrated because I longed to wear this dress, and there it was as if I could not hide it.

I took some leg foundation to cover it, but it was of no use. I felt annoyed that I had to look for another outfit and wear pants I usually hate, but now I had no choice.

I even remember the exact words he said to me, "I haven't seen you wearing pants for a long time?" Then it hit me. I have to do something about these stretch marks!

Chapter 3:
How I Looked for Remedies

Many mothers-to-be say they want to avoid stretch marks again, but it is much more complicated than that. You can't always prevent them from happening, or it will get worse. So many women suffer because of the pressure and guilt they put on themselves.

Most women worry about the perks of being a new mom, and they always have many concerns about it. It's not your fault! Just take care of yourself during pregnancy and be happy.

Moisturizing regularly with cocoa butter or almond oil helps prevent dryness after pregnancy; this prevents stretch marks from forming because preventative measures avoid the skin from drying up during pregnancy and prevent fine lines.

You can also look online and find amazing facts about over-the-counter products to help you deal with them. Asking for professional help is also one of the best ways to be well aware of the best thing to do.

Facts that can help inform you in this aspect can be a mind opener, and later on, you can share them with friends or women who share the same dilemma you've been through during the pregnancy phase.

Prolonged side sleeping is the best way to prevent stretch marks. Side sleepers have less belly fat and better circulation, which means they're less likely than other people to develop those ugly lines of dried skin that occur during pregnancy!

The benefits don't stop there - getting a tummy tuck at the end of pregnancy can also help you avoid future problems like wrinkles or sagging breasts too. It is sometimes very frustrating to think about the consequences of being pregnant and becoming a mother, but I am happy despite all this. I know most women can relate to my opinion, and all we have to do is embrace motherhood and take care of ourselves.

Pregnancy is a tough time for your body. It's not surprising that many women want to take preventative measures against the harsh realities of aging- such as stretch marks and sagging skin due just from the pregnancy itself!

Working moms, to be exact, are very conscious when it comes to this. And there is nothing wrong with it; all of us just wanted to stay in shape and still look good.

Finding ways to care for ourselves is not a sin; we want to be back in form and look suitable for our partner. Exercising after you give birth will help keep those pesky lines at bay before they can form on more vulnerable areas like thighs or arms. It keeps us fit and healthy.

In addition, exercise has been shown over recent years to reduce resting heart rate and blood pressure, among other positive effects, which mean less stress attached directly onto baby-making moments in their lives. Most pregnant women are encouraged to do simple exercises that are good for their health and the baby.

Your doctor's advice to eat healthy with the help of activity can be efficient. After giving birth, regular exercise can prevent many life-threatening diseases, relieve stress, make you healthy, and help you get back on your feet and enjoy motherhood. It is also a way to enjoy a healthy life with your family.

Docosahexaenoic acid or DHA can help your body get vitamins and nutrients that will keep the stretch marks from happening. Moisturizing with cocoa butter, almond oil, or other substances can keep it from happening. Some women

Cocoa butter is a natural, effective way to prevent stretch marks during pregnancy and help avoid the appearance of fine lines. It's not just for your belly! You can also use cocoa butter as protection against sun damage on other areas like arms or legs when they're exposed most often in summer weather.

Stretch marks are caused by hormonal changes in your body when you are pregnant. Preventing stretch marks with preventative measures helps avoid the stretching of the skin during your pregnancy and contains fine lines. Breastfeeding is a preventative measure to prevent stretch marks because preventive measures prevent the skin from forming during pregnancy and prevent fine lines.

You may have heard that stretch marks are forms of scar tissue and a sign of puberty, but they're reddish lines on the skin brought about by sudden size changes to the body. Stretch mark prevention during adolescence with cocoa butter can help keep your breasts smooth! It's also wise to take care of yourself- after giving birth or while pregnant--to ensure beautiful skin for years.

Chapter 4:
How I Get Rid of Stretch Marks After Pregnancy Without Scaring Myself

The most helpful prevention measure I employed was wearing black tights every day when it got too hot outside. It helped avoid my skin getting irritated by the warm weather and prevented any stretch marks from showing up on their way.

When you look in a mirror, what do you see? Not a reflection of your true self, but rather the image of a woman constantly consumed by her body. We are always judged as we walk through life, criticized as we encounter people who disapprove of our bodies and are frequently let down by those, we seek comfort from in our lives.

Our society continually puts women in these boxes and creates false ideals that not everybody can replicate; it's nearly impossible.

My stretch marks are in the worst possible places: on my stomach and legs. They are unsightly, but thankfully stretch marks can prevent them with a bit of ingenuity! For years after having four children, I would worry about whether or not these dark bars of skin were going away anytime soon.

Until one day, an acquaintance came up to me at work without realizing what she said, "Hey, how did you get rid of that ugly striking?" Bingo - that's right, there is nothing more satisfying than beating your body into submission just because society tells us it's wrong to overpower ourselves physically afterward.

I took preventative measures to prevent stretch marks during pregnancy on her legs because it was difficult to prevent stretch marks on her stomach. Her preventive measures included wearing tight pants, skirts, and tights during pregnancy and covering her legs with clothes in hot weather, even in the summertime.

Chapter 5:
Healthy Tips to Prevent Stretch Marks

I'm a young mom, and I have many stretch marks on my stomach after pregnancy. If you are also struggling with the same issue, then don't feel so alone! Most of us share the same problem. One of the most helpful things you can do to prevent stretch marks, whether pregnant or not, is maintaining a healthy weight. Let's stop them together by following some easy steps:

1. Exercise to prevent your skin from overstretching

It's not always easy being pregnant! One of the scariest parts can be all those stretch marks that form across one's stomach during childbirth. Luckily, you'll only need to worry about this if preventative measures aren't taken in advance- but why wait? Exercises like swimming or yoga are perfect choices because they help maintain blood circulation and give your skin much-needed support from too much moisture drying out on top of it and who doesn't want toned arms while planking?

2. Eat Healthy Fats to prevent stretch marks.

Healthy fats like olive oil, peanuts, and avocados will keep you looking toned. But it's not just about what we eat - it also matters how much water is in our bodies when these cells change shape to form stretch marks for a boy or girl!

The best way to avoid them? Drink lots of fluids (at least two glasses per day) so that less sodium builds up on skin surfaces; try my favorite drink: lemon juice mixed with warm honey as an easy-peasy natural remedy during hot summer months.

3. Maintain Proper Hydration to prevent stretch marks

A good drink can do wonders for helping combat these issues, so I recommend staying topped off with H2O throughout each day if possible (even while working/ exercising).

Additionally, I highly recommend staying away from any caffeinated beverages (coffee, soda, and other drinks.). At the same time, pregnant - caffeine can pass through the placenta into your baby's bloodstream if you need coffee or soda that badly, limit yourself to one cup per day but only if it won't affect your sleeping pattern (which, of course, it might, so if you do, feel free to have your one cup).

Caffeine isn't the only thing that can affect your sleep while pregnant. Try to eliminate any distractions in the bedroom, such as overly bright lights, loud noises, and pets.

4. Apply Vitamin E oil on your stomach daily

I don't know about you, but I'm always looking for a way to keep my skin from stretching. You might think that only celebrities have stretch marks in their childhood photos and movies from when they were supermodels-but now we all want better bodies!

Luckily, we have vitamin E, which prevents these unwanted scars by strengthening the elasticity of our tissue. So, even if something does happen later, like weight gain or pregnancy (or both), it won't be enough time has passed yet for those ugly tones on your stomach to show up as well.

The natural ingredient will minimize them significantly while improving other cosmetic imperfections such as fine lines around the eye area. This nutrient helps deliver oxygen deep into dermal layers where wound healing starts.

5. Eat enough protein to prevent Pregnancy Stretch Marks

Protein is essential for muscle growth, so it's necessary to take enough during pregnancy. Your baby needs protein too! Don't forget to eat lean meat and fish or eggs from happy chickens who get fed their natural diet of good bug juice (namely soybeans), dairy products made with whole milk instead of skimmed liters like there's no tomorrow--and donuts?

Of course not; those are just as bad if you're trying to avoid gaining weight while pregnant but still maintaining your taste buds because nothing beats a homemade doughnut on cold mornings or afternoons either come daylight savings time has done its thing.

Stretching your skin to accommodate a growing baby is just part of pregnancy. However, if you prevent stretch marks from forming in the first place by applying Revitol Scar Cream, then it can be good news!

Suppose you already have them on hand, however. In that case, this product also works wonders for getting rid of those unsightly dark rings around slim fingers and ankles after surgery/injury recovery periods.

The biggest problem with being pregnant isn't only that our bodies change drastically (which they should). Still, sadly enough, sometimes bad things happen like accidents or something else that might trigger us into developing new scars all over again, even when we thought everything had healed entirely back.

The best way you can treat and prevent stretch marks is with cream. The critical thing you need while growing during pregnancy and after giving birth is hydration!

Being hydrated is a key to healthy glowing skin.

The more you take fluids, the more your skin will be flawless. It gives you a chance not to acquire stretch marks, and it is also beneficial for you and your baby.

There are so many products that are available for your skin. You can purchase it online, or some are available in groceries, convenience stores, and drug stores. It is also wise to seek professional help, or maybe you can read some information over a magazine or advertisements that are within your reach.

Just make sure to talk to your doctor about it for the safety of your baby too. Never hesitate to ask if you are very much concerned about it. Always remember to put the health of your baby first and foremost. Although some are very safe to use, always ensure that it will not affect your baby if you use some products.

Applying this topical treatment will keep your skin moisturized so that it has elasticity when needed most, which helps avoid those ugly scars on the abdomen area from all of our suitcase's expansion process known in polite company as "growing up."

Growing a human in your belly is a remarkable phenomenon. As our human body goes through a wide variety of changes in the process, sensory to hormonal, circulatory to physical, but the easiest to identify and track is the size of your stomach. Stretch marks are most common during pregnancy, and that is reality.

However, it's okay if some women like me have a strong desire to prevent them. We know that there are plenty of creams available anywhere, but we have to make sure that it is safe for both the mother and the child. Using a stretch mark cream may not prevent or eliminate stretch marks, but it might help make them less pronounced and noticeable by improving skin elasticity and giving you smoother skin.

Plus, using stretch mark cream can be a fantastic way to get in touch with your body and give yourself some tender loving care throughout your pregnancy. It is not harmful to take care of your body, and it is very therapeutic for you and the baby.

There is an array of products you can choose from the pharmacy or online. You can also look for some products that you can use on your do-it-your own remedies.

Certain ingredients like:

- Nut butter which you can find in cocoa, shea, or jojoba.
- Vitamins that are rich in A and E
- Hyaluronic acid
- Coconut, argan, or rosehip oil
- Aloe vera
- Peptides

You can make your own if you think it will be best for you as long as you use the safest ingredients there are. Finding a little information about what to do is normal, and it is somehow very informative, and the more information you have, the more it is safe.

There are so many products that give promising results. You can buy some cheap products or whatever that can convince you to give good results like Revitol. This product is clinically proven to be effective. Aside from using products for your stretch marks, avoid scratching your skin if you feel itchy. It can worsen and deepen the area of your stretch marks.

You may also experience a burning sensation caused by tiny blood vessels, and it can cause the skin to break. You must refrain from stretching any affected area for your skin's sake.

Here are some simple tips for you to help reduce stretch marks;

- Eat food rich in Omega 3s.
- Gain a healthy amount of weight during pregnancy.
- Use a moisturizer all the time.

- Avoid anabolic steroid use.
- Get vitamin D.
- Limit or avoid steroids cream for itching.

Chapter 6:
Why Stretch Marks Happen

Stretch marks are often the results of a rapid increase in your body size.

But some are also caused by medical conditions, including:

Diabetes- Most people with Diabetes often gain and lose weight intensely. So, they are most likely to develop stretch marks due to it.

Obesity: Apart from getting pregnant, obesity can cause stretch marks that appear in some body parts. It mainly stretches the skin to its limit if one gains much weight.

Cushing disease- Changes to the amount and distribution of body fat, decreased muscle mass leading to weakness and reduced stamina, thinning skin can cause stretch marks.

However, the condition itself does not cause stretch marks. Instead, the weight gain or body size increase usually results in stretch marks appearing in your body.

A growth spurt is another cause when your child has a more intense period of growth; during this time, they may want to eat more and change their sleeping habits, thus increasing their body size. Growth spurts are very common in teenage boys. They often increase appetite, improve bone and muscle growth, and also cause stretch marks to appear.

You are picking up a significant amount of weight. Make some changes so that you can lose some weight. Educate yourself by eating healthy food or creating your diet, like eating more high-fiber food to lose weight. Have discipline and watch you eat.

You are putting on a large amount of muscle mass. Drink plenty of water to help you build your muscle mass. Eat more food that is rich in protein to boost your muscle mass. Building muscles requires positive energy balance; working out and eating the right food can help you. Look for a program that will help you or seek professional help.

You are experiencing significant swelling or growth in one area. These can include pregnancy stretch marks and injury stretch marks. If your skin experiences some swelling due to injury or pregnancy, it can be more prone to stretch marks.

Most people question: "Does losing weight get rid of stretch marks"? If stretch marks do not go away on their own or at least fade to the point that they are no longer noticeable, it means that the chances of the damage in your skin are too deep. It also means that it will be tough for you to get rid of it.

Taking care of yourself, especially your skin can lessen the development or traces of stretch marks. It is common for men and women who lose weight. Having significant structures or being fat and losing weight can be harsh to your skin, and you can be very prone to this.

As long as you are well informed and ask for professional help, you can answer this question yourself. Just exercise, eat healthily, and you can use products to lighten the traces of your stretch marks.

Many products on the market can repair your skin or fade away stretch marks. Some even use over-the-counter creams, lotion, or any soap that can help you lighten up the traces of your stretch marks. There are cases that it goes away, but there are some that it is hard to get rid of and take time.

You can also use alternative ways like herbal products or do it with your natural ingredients like Aloe vera or coconut oil. These can help in your dilemma about stretch marks.

"Why Do Skin Changes After Gain and Weight loss?" When weight is gained, the body increases in size, which in turn causes the skin to follow suit. It means that the more you gain weight, the more your skin stretches and tends to develop stretch marks as you lose weight.

This scenario is prevalent in women who get pregnant. As the baby grows to the woman's belly, she will gain weight, as well as the skin in her belly area, avoid will most likely stretch to its maximum limit. You can have stretch marks in any part of your body, but they are most common on your stomach, breast area, upper arms, thighs, and buttocks.

These areas in our body often tend to become big and, even worse, get huge depending on whether we gain weight or become pregnant. Many women experiences stretch marks during pregnancy as the skin stretches numerous ways to make room for the baby. This continual tugging and stretching can cause the unwanted

stretch marks.

It also appears to teenagers because of sudden growth or changes in their bodily appearance. It mostly seems to those who gain or lose weight at a specific time.

Teenagers nowadays are very conscious of their outer appearance.

It is a must for them to look good, and some work out hard and lose weight, or some gain weight to look for them to look good; here come stretch marks. The next thing they know is that it's all in there, and they may think it's the worst thing that happens to them.

Most of them don't know about losing or gaining weight, so they are most prone to it aside from pregnant women. So, for me, it is better to educate them about it and inform them about the things they need to know about how to prevent it or how to take care of their skin. Prevention is better than curing or minimizing. It is like taking care of it before it happens.

Chapter 7:
How to Remove Stretch Marks for Good

Pregnancy is a good time for women. But it can have problems too, like stretch marks. Studies show that around 90% of all pregnant women get them. This mark is because the skin needs to stretch without scarring too deeply into the surrounding skin.

The best way to get rid of pregnancy stretch marks is with hydroquinone or retinol cream. These ingredients increase production in collagen, which fades the color over time as it produces new cells and sloughs off old ones left behind on your skin from previous scars - even if they're still visible now!

Home remedies and doctor-prescribed treatments may help diminish the appearance of stretch marks. Collagen is a protein underneath your skin that makes it more elastic and supports your skin.

Your skin tries to heal any abrupt changes or tear in your skin collagen. With the proper treatment like Retinol or other products, it will help you bring your skin back. Don't forget to exfoliate your skin and pamper it once in a while.

Getting rid of stretch marks in a completely natural way can help too. The proper exercise and food intake help your skin to heal and replenish itself.

These remedies will help minimize the appearance of stretch marks and help them to fade more quickly. You can also use a topical extract of vitamin A, or take vitamin A orally, which can make a difference to your skin's health and overall appearance.

Don't forget to include in your diet rich in vitamin A such as carrots and sweet potatoes.

Some also use or rub a sugar scrub on the skin to exfoliate your damaged area. A Dermatologist performs Microdermabrasion, and it is a proven method to make stretch marks fade away.

You can also do it in your way by mixing your mixture. Here's how you can do it:

- Mix one cup sugar with ¼ cup of softening agents like coconut oil or almond oil.
- Mix it well until it reaches the consistency of wet and grainy sand.
- Add a little freshly squeezed lemon juice.
- Scrub the mixture on the specific part of your body where the stretch marks are visible.
- Repeat several times in a week or while taking a shower. Do the scrub in 8 to 10 minutes.

Aloe Vera is also helpful to your skin. It has its natural ingredient that will heal your skin soft too. You can use it daily after taking a shower.

Hyaluronic acid can also help you. It is available in your collagen products like soap and lotion. Some products have it, or you can take it orally. It will allow your skin to keep it in shape and will appear healthy.

Coconut oil is considered one of the best home remedies too. Its healing properties can help you get rid of stretch marks quickly. Applying Virgin Coconut oil to your skin at least once a day will give you glowing skin, help reduce your skin abnormalities, and help take away stretch marks for good.

Some other treatments like Laser therapy, needling, and Microdermabrasion are three clinical treatments for stretch marks.

1. Microdermabrasion involves exfoliating the skin. It improves the appearance of stretch marks.

2. Needling is a new treatment in which collagen is injected underneath the top layer of your skin. This process is very effective too.

Stretch marks have the possibility of fading over time until it becomes barely noticeable. Women who develop stretch marks in pregnancy become less-prominent in some areas in around 6 to 12 months.

It never goes away that easily but may reduce the stretch marks appearance with treatments available at the palm of your hand. All you have to do is learn how to take care of your skin and do something about it, and it will solve your problems in no time at all.

For me, the best treatment for stretch marks is prevention. Always keep your skin hydrated, moisturize it with proper creams rich in natural ingredients like coconut oil, eat healthily, and exercise more.

Self-care is the best care that you will reward yourself. Now the real question is can you make it all go away? Does losing weight get rid of your stretch marks? Can women still have a chance of having flawless, stretch effects-free skin?

Conclusion

Pregnancy is the best gift a woman can get. It comes with many perks, of course, long-term agonies, painful delivery, and hours of labor, and being a mother is not that easy. It is like fulfilling a woman's dream, and it is, of course, the true essence of a woman.

After delivery, here comes the reality: being pregnant makes many changes to a woman's body. We gain weight. Of course, after delivery, some women lose weight and regain their body back. So here goes the stretch marks that leave traces in most parts of our bodies.

It is an agony for some women, especially those working and very conscious of how they look. Some women take it seriously, and for them, it is a big deal, so they will do whatever it takes to deal with stretch marks and must take a step to let it all go away.

Pregnancy can be an opportunity for self-care, whether you want to make your skin more elastic or avoid stretch marks. It's not all bad news! I hope this book has helped teach you about the science behind these problems and how they may affect your body during pregnancy.

Pregnancy is often when many women are looking to care for themselves - so take advantage of it by using some of these stretches, oils, vitamins, and nutrients that worked well for me if there are any other questions on what's safe or harmful during pregnancy.

For me, being a mother is great and all that goes with it. It is essential as long as you know how to take care of your body after giving birth. Don't let pregnancy change the way you look; it is not a crime that all you want is to be as attractive and flawless to others and your husband, of course.

There is nothing wrong with that. Pampering our skin is the best self-care for us mothers. Motherhood is a privilege, and being a woman who takes care of herself is a gift of happiness for us. Enjoy being a mother and being a woman.

Whether you developed stretch marks due to pregnancy or to reasons like gaining and losing weight, you have the authority to search for standard information or to ask professional help. After all, it is your body; you ought to take care of it and do something about it.

Skin is the mantle of our outer appearance; if you are a person or a woman conscious about your outward appearance, you have to look for ways to eliminate this kind of problem. Career-oriented men and women of a certain age that usually make a living out of their looks like Models, Actors, and actresses, or those who face people most of the time must take care of their skin.

It is customary and required, so there is nothing wrong if most of them take stretch marks seriously. Suppose we familiar people worry about it, how much more to them. Taking care of ourselves is not a crime, you know, we must learn to love ourselves by taking care of it.

We owe ourselves to be pampered, spoiled once in a while, and mostly, our skin is the most common thing we worry about all the time. Having glowing, flawless, and healthy skin makes us confident and sexy. It gives us inner confidence in the beauty that reflects in our outer appearance. It makes us happy and content.

We were able to get you a trial bottle of Revitol Stretchmark Cream only at https://bit.ly/zulu80

SCAN ME

www.ingramcontent.com/pod-product-compliance
Lightning Source LLC
Chambersburg PA
CBHW022107020426
42335CB00012B/864